PRESCRIPTIONS
FOR
LIFE WITH CANCER

Dr. Eric Fairbank

Illustrations by Boré Hoekstra

Hill of Content

FOREWORD

It is possible that to write a booklet such as this is the height of audacity.

How can someone who is just a GP, with no personal experience of cancer, be prescribing this approach to a life threatening illness?

Out of context some may find it all rather off-putting and feel like asking "How can he know what it's like and tell me what to do?"

What then is my excuse?

Life is not endless. Cancer underlines this and creates a sense of urgency.

Minds more perceptive than mine, professionals more qualified and people with personal experience of cancer have all written on this topic. Wisdom abounds, but is often scattered or almost hidden from the average reader in bigger books, or so it seems to me.

To meet the urgency of the situation I have attempted to summarise in succinct form the collective wisdom of many others.

My choice of material is no doubt tempered by my own values and experience of life which includes over twenty five years in General Practice, the last ten involved with education groups for people with cancer and their families.

My plea is for the reader not to look upon these prescriptions as my orders, but rather as a collection of suggestions that I think might be worth trying out for size.

Eric Fairbank

PRESCRIPTIONS FOR LIFE WITH CANCER

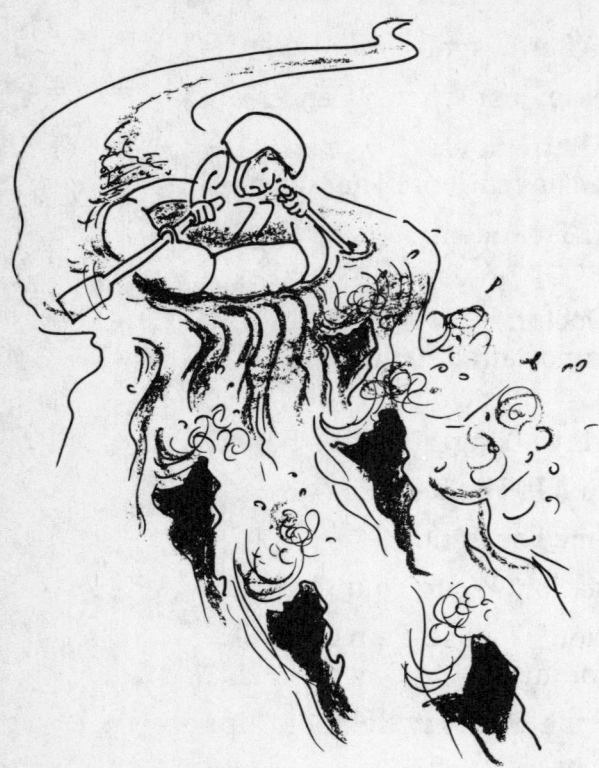

After a diagnosis of cancer, life will never be the same again.

It will be different in many ways - more worrying, more challenging, perhaps even more rewarding - but never quite the same. One of the more frightening aspects is the feeling of loss of control and helplessness with no guarantee of survival.

Stories abound concerning the various treatments and their side effects and there is the constant fear of spread or recurrence. All of this turns life upside down - not only for the person with cancer but also family and friends.

Cancer is a life threatening illness and successful coping means not only adapting to the disease itself but also to the alterations in life brought about by the disease. One of the central problems is living constantly with uncertainty and a permanent feeling of insecurity. Time frames can only be expressed as probabilities.

Yet it is worth remembering that half of all people diagnosed with cancer will survive. They will have overcome such common psychological reactions as disbelief and denial, anger, blame and guilt and dealt with the fears of isolation, vulnerability and mutilation. They will have acknowledged the seriousness of cancer, faced up to reality and then realized that things can be done.

Coping with cancer has been compared with rafting down a river. While the ultimate direction is determined (it's no good rowing upstream) manoeuvring the raft to avoid disastrous collisions is possible so that the trip can end safely

The best results in cancer treatment are obtained when the patient's own very real resources of mind and will and spirit complement the efforts of the physician, surgeon and radiotherapist. It is possible to re-establish some control while living with day to day stresses and adjusting plans for the future as well. For those in whom cancer cannot be eliminated, aim to live well, perhaps even better, accepting, but not yielding to the illness.

Every experience of life threatening illness is distinct and individual responses are very different. There is much more to cancer besides its physical aspects. It also means dealing with mental and spiritual stresses of the past, present and future. It means walking down the path that confronts the meaning of illness, of life and of death.

Hopefully this booklet will be something of a map, it's chapters worthy of sign posts to guide you on the journey.

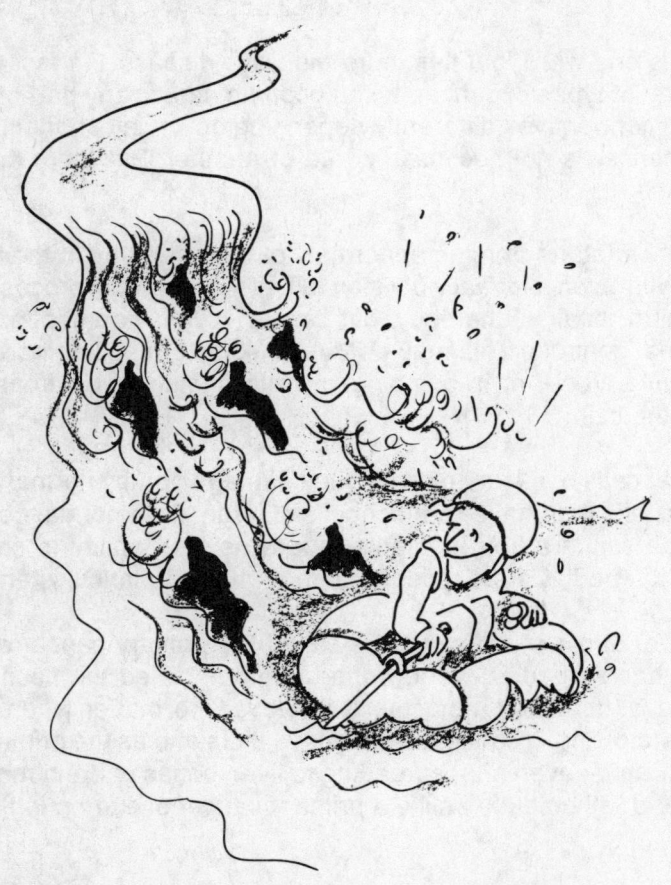

KNOW YOUR DISEASE: JUST WHAT IS CANCER?

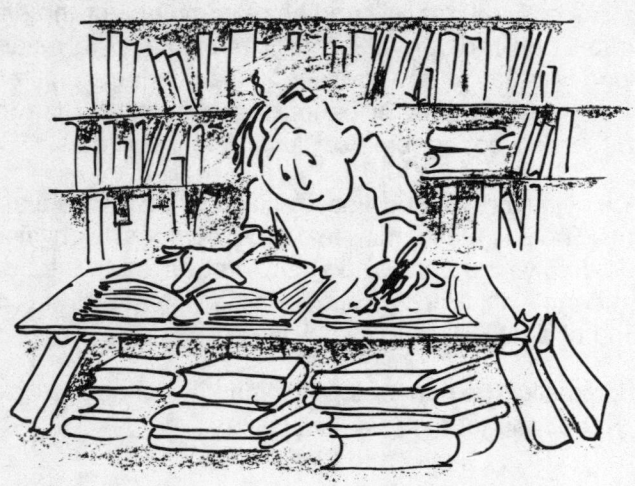

Cancer is one word, but it is more than one disease. In fact there are over 200 different types of cancer. It can occur in almost any part of the body and each cancer behaves differently depending on its cell of origin. What is true of one cancer is not necessarily true of another. But there are some basic similarities.

Each cancer starts from an abnormal cell whether it be in the breast, bowel, lung or wherever. Normally division of cells is a healthy process essential for growth and repair of the body, but cancer cells divide haphazardly, outside the normal controls. This may be due to some genetic defect inside the cell itself acting alone, or in combination with damaging environmental factors outside the cell.

As cancer cells continue to divide they damage nearby normal cells. Another characteristic that makes cancer cells different from normal cells (and which separates cancers from benign tumours) is their ability to spread to other parts of the body via the blood stream or the lymphatic system.

The site of origin of the cancer is called the primary cancer and the site to which it has spread eg. liver, bones, brain is called the secondary cancer. The process is called metastasis. However, no matter where a secondary cancer is growing, it continues to behave the same as the primary cancer. So a breast cancer even after spreading to liver, bones or brain remains a breast cancer and will be quite unlike a primary cancer occurring in those organs.

WHY CANCER CAUSES HARM

Cancer therefore causes harm by damaging normal cells at the primary or secondary site. Cancer cells may also secrete harmful hormones which contribute to poor appetite and weight loss. Further harm to the body may occur through various biochemical changes and infections eg. pneumonia. Development of blood clots occurs in some cases while bleeding tendencies occur in others.

TYPES OF CANCER

The different types of cancer may be broadly divided into two groups - the solid cancers and the blood forming cancers.

Solid cancers are either carcinomas (85%) or sarcomas. Carcinomas include cancers of the breast, bowel, lung, prostate and skin while sarcomas occur in muscles, bones and connective tissues.

Blood forming cancers include leukaemia (over production of various abnormal white cells), myeloma (from bone-marrow cells called plasma cells), and lymphoma (from cells in the lymphatic system).

CAUSES OF CANCER

While cancer can occur at any age most cancers are diagnosed in men and women over 55 years of age. Nearly one person in three will experience it in one form or another by the age of 75. It is not always possible to define the exact cause of a cancer (there may be multiple causes) but in over 70% of cases it is thought that the environment plays a role. Smoking, a diet high in fat, too much exposure to sunshine, occupational hazards - asbestos, harmful chemicals, radiation and probably stress all play a significant part in triggering the abnormal division of cells leading to cancer. It is important to note that it is not contagious.

Some types of cancer do have a tendency to run in families eg. breast and bowel and knowledge of this may be important in its early detection, so important to a successful outcome.

THE DIAGNOSIS

Because of the variety of cancers there is no one simple test to diagnose them all. The ease of diagnosis depends to a large extent on the site of origin - a visible skin cancer is more readily detected than a hidden bowel cancer, when warning signs may not be specific.

Screening tests on people with no symptoms are designed to diagnose cancer in its early stages eg. pap smear, mammography.

Blood tests rarely make a definite diagnosis except in leukaemia.

Many tests are available to assist in diagnosis from Xrays, CAT scans, Ultrasound to more invasive procedures such as colonoscopy (examination of the large bowel), bronchoscopy (respiratory system) and laparoscopy (abdominal cavity). The bottom line is that for accurate diagnosis a sample of cells needs to be examined under the microscope. Cells can be obtained from a piece of solid tissue removed at operation (biopsy) from a scraping of cells or aspiration of cells through a fine needle (cytology).

In addition to diagnosing the type of cancer it is also important to determine the extent of the spread i.e. the stage of the cancer, as this will have a bearing on deciding the most appropriate form of treatment. Sometimes the cancer is at an advanced stage before the diagnosis is made and it may be difficult to find the primary site. Nevertheless appropriate treatment can be planned.

CONSIDER THE ALTERNATIVES: ORTHODOX AND UNCONVENTIONAL THERAPIES

The person with cancer, feeling isolated and under pressure, often feels that there is no choice but to accept whatever treatment is offered and hope for the best.

However, even with the vast knowledge of medical science at his/her disposal it is questionable that one doctor should dictate what sort of treatment a person with a certain type of cancer must have for a successful outcome. Remarkable differences exist in the way cancer is treated in various advanced countries and differences also occur between surgeons, radiotherapists and oncologists (physicians who specialise in cancer) - each tending to favour the contribution of their own speciality. (It has been likened to the debate about the relative merits of the Army, Airforce and Navy!)

For the patient who wants to be involved in treatment decisions there is a need to overcome their ignorance about cancer. Information can be gathered from a number of sources. It is every person's right to seek a second opinion which can be co-ordinated by your general practitioner. Seeing an oncologist in advance of surgery is often a wise move to become more aware of choices a surgeon may not fully explain.

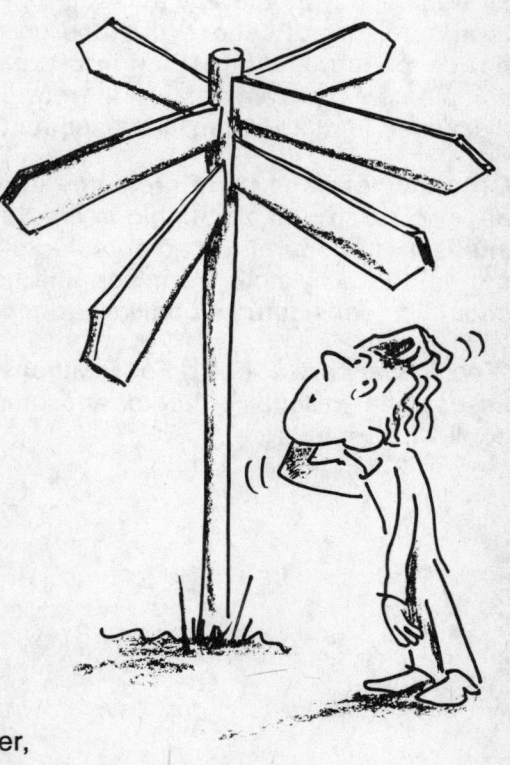

Someone - yourself or a support person - who is willing and able to read medical literature can make a big difference in your ability to make informed choices. Relevant material can be obtained at a medical or local hospital library. Even buying a medical dictionary may be worthwhile. Some excellent resource books are available, one of the better ones being "Your Cancer, Your Life" by Dr. Trish Reynolds.

Along with basic information concerning surgery, radiotherapy and chemotherapy, it encourages (with practical examples), the questions to ask concerning the relative benefits and risks associated with a particular course of action.

UNCONVENTIONAL TREATMENTS

Rather than too few choices, sometimes there are too many. Unconventional treatments include some of the best and some of the worst treatments available.

The best involve the person in his own treatment, promote health and improve quality of life. They are complementary to orthodox treatment and give some control back to the individual who generally does not regret having undertaken them, whatever the outcome.

Such approaches include meditation, attention to diet, vitamin and mineral supplementation, exercise, massage, support groups, positive thinking strategies, psychotherapy and spiritual contemplation with prayer. Long term survivors of cancer all place great importance on meditation and peace of mind using their intuition to guide them further. Such complementary therapies are therefore to be encouraged and many are discussed in more detail in subsequent chapters.

On the other hand there are some unproven treatments which seem to offer so much that a struggle is created between the emotions and the intellect. In general, treatments that claim to cope with all cancers, that are said to be simple, harmless and non toxic, that are also expensive should be considered as unlikely to meet expectations.

"Facing Cancer - Looking For Solutions" by Liz Byrski gives an objective assessment of both orthodox and unconventional treatments and is a book worth reading.

UNDERSTAND YOUR TREATMENT: SURGERY, RADIOTHERAPY, CHEMOTHERAPY

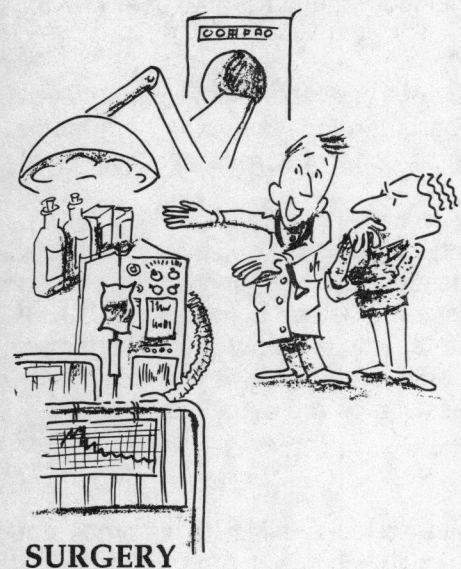

Many cancers can be successfully treated.

The main methods for treating cancer are surgery (operating to remove cancerous tissue), radiotherapy (destroying cancer cells with high energy radiation eg. Xrays) and chemotherapy (using drugs to destroy or inhibit cancer cells). These may be used either alone or in combination depending on such factors as the type of cancer and its stage of spread. With each of these treatments the aims may be curative or palliative - the latter aimed at controlling symptoms and improving the quality of life when the cancer is beyond cure.

SURGERY

Accessible cancers localised at the primary site may be removed at operation, along with some surrounding normal tissue. Nearby lymph glands may also be removed. Examination of the tissues removed under the microscope gives clues about local or distant spread but it is not possible to be 100% certain that metastasis has not occurred prior to the operation. Therefore follow-up is necessary and on average claims of cure should be postponed for about five years.

Palliative surgery may be used to relieve an obstruction or prevent a bone from fracturing - the aim being control of symptoms rather than cure.

RADIOTHERAPY

Like surgery, curative radiotherapy is also designed for localised cancers. Xrays produced by machines or Gamma rays from radioactive substances such as cobalt and radium kill cancer cells. Treatment is planned carefully to minimize damage to normal cells. Precisely the same region must be treated each time, sometimes with the help of a special mould made to keep parts of the body still. Rays are neither seen nor felt and in no more than a few minutes the treatment is over.

Curative radiotherapy is usually given on a daily basis spread over several weeks to allow time for normal tissues to repair. Cancers vary in their response to radiation which is used particularly for those difficult to remove surgically. Radiotherapy may also be used in combination with surgery to deal with any cancer cells perhaps surviving nearby.

Palliative radiotherapy can reduce the size of a cancer to relieve pain, prevent bleeding or ulceration and so has an important role in controlling symptoms. Such treatments may be given as a single dose of spread over just a few days.

Although radiotherapy is completely painless there may be some side effects such as tiredness and nausea or local reactions such as skin reddening similar to light sunburn. Unless the head itself is being treated hair does not fall out. Treatment does not make you radioactive so it is quite safe to be with other people. Unlike surgery radiotherapy is only available in a few specialised centres but travel and accommodation assistance are usually available.

CHEMOTHERAPY

Chemotherapy cures some cancers such as leukaemias, lymphomas and testicular tumours. It may also be used in conjunction with other treatments if there is a risk of spread or it might be used to relieve symptoms such as pain.

Anti cancer drugs may be taken orally or given intramuscularly or intravenously, sometimes via special catheters, and circulate throughout the body to destroy or inhibit growth of cancer cells wherever they may be. To maximise the anti cancer effect several drugs acting at different points of the cells life cycles are often combined.

Because normal cells, especially those that divide rapidly are also damaged there are often some side effects. However the side effects do vary according to the drugs used and from person to person. Normal tissues most affected are the stomach and intestines, hair follicles, mucous membranes and bone marrow. Common side effects are therefore nausea, vomiting and diarrhoea, hair loss, soreness of the mouth and anaemia, easy bruising and infections.

Intravenous chemotherapy sessions can last from a few hours to several days followed by a rest period of usually several weeks to allow normal tissues to recover. Blood tests taken prior to the next treatment ensure that this has happened. To make a decision whether chemotherapy (or any other treatment) is for you, it is a matter of asking enough questions to be sufficiently informed and able to weigh up the potential benefits against the likely risks.

HORMONE TREATMENTS

Some cancers are sensitive to hormones and so control may be sought either by giving hormones or surgically removing glands that produce hormones.

The breast and prostate provide the best examples of hormone dependent cancers. Antioestrogen tablets control breast cancer whereas surgical or chemical castration or taking oestrogen tablets are used to control cancer of the prostate.

IMMUNOTHERAPY

Immunotherapy seeks to boost the immune system's ability to fight cancer cells though not all cancers produce a good immune response in the body. Natural substances such as interferon are used in this way particularly in leukaemias and lymphomas.

Research is being directed towards developing antibodies against certain types of cancer cells. More detail about these treatments or other more specialised procedures such as bone marrow transplantation may be obtained from Anti Cancer Council publications.

DIAGNOSE YOUR DOCTOR:
DEVELOPING AN IMPORTANT RELATIONSHIP

Taking time to make the right choice of doctor is a good investment. Pay at least as much attention to it as choosing a car!

Like any relationship a good doctor-patient relationship depends on communication, which is a two-way street. In diagnosing your doctor you may therefore need to check that the traditional relationship of power and knowledge on the one hand and dependence and submission on the other has been modified to allow for your participation in conversations and medical decisions.

Friends and neighbours, other patients, other doctors and nurses can all help you make a choice to ensure that you will be a partner in the management of your disease.

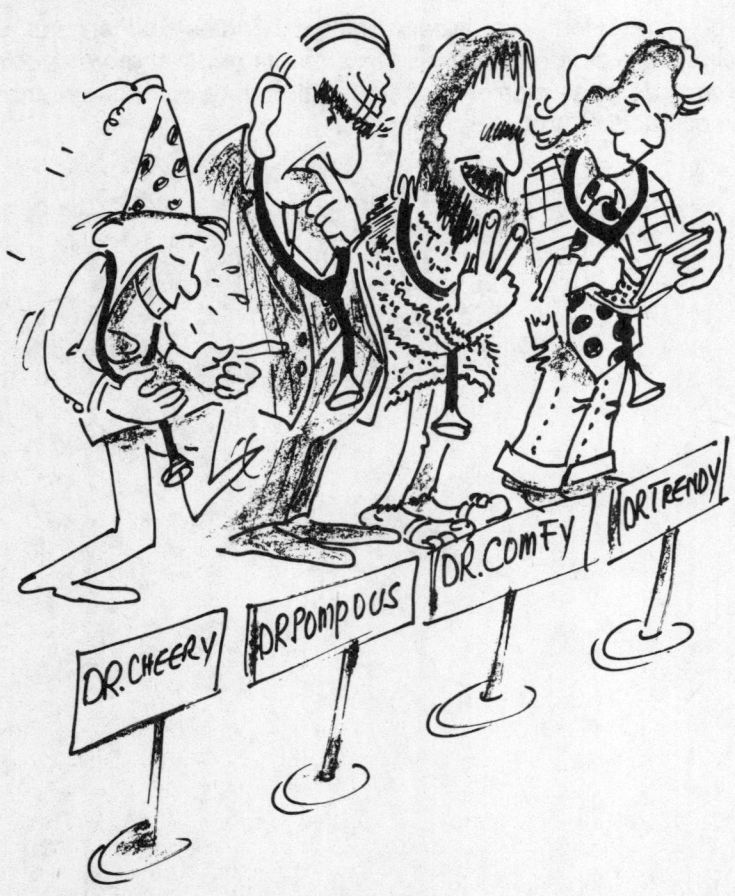

On the other hand you may prefer a more direct approach and make an appointment to find out for yourself. In many busy practices you can accept appointments with all the doctors in turn until you find the one you are happiest with, then see that particular doctor in future. Use your senses to check whether or not your doctor is with you emotionally. Is he/she paying attention to the right issues with the right words? Do you think that your relationship might be damaged by the progression of your disease when serious illness often highlights doctors' limitations? Different doctors may handle different stages of the disease better.

Different doctors also suit different personalities. Do you prefer a Dr. Cheery (healthy and optimistic) or Dr. Pompous (in a formal suit) or Dr. Comfy (in a hand knitted cardigan)? Dr. Trendy wears coloured shirts and funny ties and has all the latest information - or so it seems. With a little luck however you may find your Dr. Perfect who listens, meets your eye, achieves immediate rapport, is humane, helpful and interested, and makes you feel better whether or not you get a prescription.

Once diagnosed and chosen, establish a good working relationship with your doctor by keeping up your end of the communication. Be prepared for a consultation with your symptoms loud and clear in your mind. Write down any questions you have and get to the point by expressing your underlying concerns. Doctors will always snap into action if you say "I'm worried about this lump or discharge, or my tummy - could you have a look at it please and put my mind at rest?"

Do not withhold information out of fear of hearing things you really do not want to hear. Bad news now is better than worse news later. If necessary practice gentle assertion and do not be frightened to ask for a second opinion if you still feel concerned. At times having a family member or friend with you to listen in will help you with later discussions and decisions.

You should be able to come away from a doctor's consultation knowing what is wrong or what will be done to find out, what is the recommended treatment - its effects and side effects and whether there are any alternatives. Better understanding of your illness is all part of being more responsible for your own health, leads to more control and in the long run - better health.

FACE REALITY:
DO YOU HAVE TO LIVE LONGER TO LIVE BETTER?

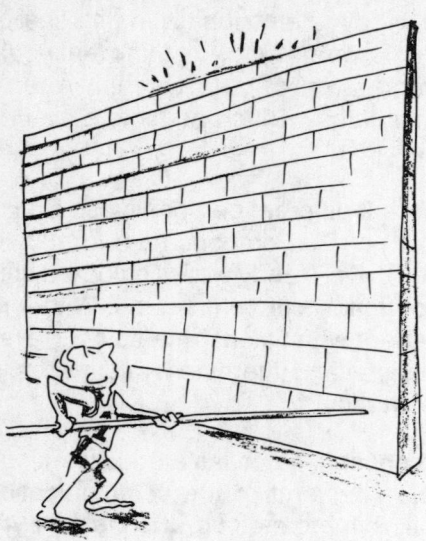

For many people cancer becomes a chronic illness. Unable to claim a cure because of the risk of recurrence or spread, there is still much living yet to be done. However, at this stage aggressive cancer treatment is likely to have taken its toll with surgery, radiotherapy and/or chemotherapy sometimes seeming to cause more illness or discomfort than the initial disease. Feeling worse now than at the time of diagnosis it's difficult to be optimistic and plan strategies for the future. Anxiety and uncertainty can be quite overwhelming.

There is a new personal time scale - B.C. (before cancer) and A.D. (after diagnosis). Each day has its ups and downs with alternating feelings, fear and frustrations at slow improvement, sleep problems, mad thoughts, self pity, even despair. Being human means complicated, unacceptable emotions - none of us is immune. It may feel like coming up against a brick wall.

However, sooner or later decisions have to be made about living with this chronic illness. This may be the time to stop and consider the question "why me?" perhaps previously raised in anger. It is often helpful to understand that we are part of a dynamic process which responds to both positive and negative influences. Perhaps by identifying and dealing with negative influences there is some chance of return to health. Looking for meaning - not to assign blame or feel guilty - but to understand, is a worthwhile pursuit.

Cancer gives the opportunity for reassessment. Am I content? Do I still want to be like, feel like that? Is it time for a change? Perhaps the question should not be "why me?" but "why now?" Look at cancer in the context of the whole of life's experiences and probably a combination of factors has led to this chronic degenerative illness.

There is no doubt that the capacity to cope is enhanced by the ability to identify, examine and discuss feelings effectively. Perhaps this is why groups of cancer patients meeting together are so effective in prolonging survival time - in fact, doubling it (Spiegel, 1993). By facing directly the threat posed by the illness and increasing social support, groups demonstrate the positive link with health and that psychological interventions have physical consequences.

Facing bad possibilities does not convert them into bad probabilities. Rather it helps people to separate such emotions as fear from anger, to see their tendency to overlap and aggravate each other. Facing reality can encourage people to regain control in their lives, to reorganise priorities, to gain new perspectives with the focus on living better not longer. Time acquires its true value when we recognize that it is not infinite.

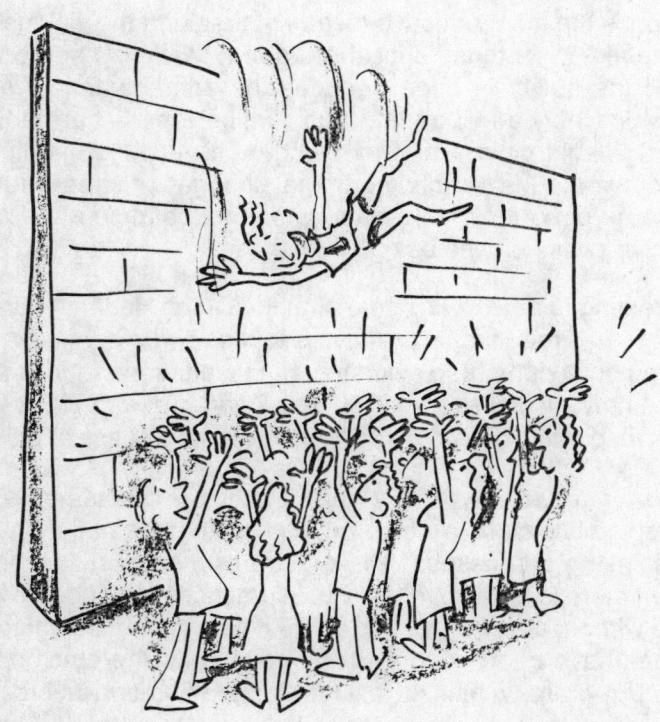

BE STILL: MEDITATION IS THE KEY

Having cancer is a stressful experience which does nothing but further impair quality of life. Appropriate psychological support is therefore essential and one of the better ways of achieving this is by including meditation as a complementary therapy.

Some argue that meditation is foreign to western cultures. Perhaps this is because our lives seem to live us, carry us along with their own crazy momentum, crammed with compulsive activity. At odd moments we tell ourselves that we should spend more time on the important things of life, but there doesn't seem to be any time left. The term "active laziness" has been used to describe this kind of busyness. To continue at this frantic pace, seeking to increase the possessions that satisfy our physical needs, will deprive us of the chance to grasp other, less tangible, but more satisfying and durable possessions.

Yet even in western cultures there can be brief moments where the mind naturally approaches the meditative state. Day dreaming, just staring out the window or being absorbed in a piece of music are moments to build on, that allow us to pause, to "be still and know".

Meditation is the most effective means of breaking the vicious circle of stress and disease. Even those critical of natural therapies agree that meditation improves the ability to cope, reduces the appreciation of pain, can make relationships between patients and families more harmonious and have beneficial effects on overall well being. The state of meditation has been shown to reverse the harmful hormonal changes of stress in the body, giving the body the opportunity to regain its natural balance and for us to achieve that elusive sense of well being.

It is interesting to note at this point that the Dutch Health Insurance Company Silvercross has reduced its premiums to those who meditate. Their decision was based on documented evidence that meditation reduces the incidence of a wide variety of diseases - 87% less heart disease, 30% less infections, 73% less respiratory disease, 49% less intestinal disease and 55% less cancer.

Meditation is a pathway to another state of consciousness - neither awake nor asleep. It is a state in which we lose awareness of the physical body and normal thinking processes. It is a state of mental stillness. In essence to meditate - there is nothing to do! But in practice many people who sit down to meditate without a technique find out just how nimble the mind can be. Many techniques have been used over the years with the common aim of stilling the mind. Progressive muscle relaxation, concentrating on breathing, mantras, listening to music and mental imagery have all been recommended.

Progressive muscle relaxation is a simple and reliable technique.

1. You should be physically still, balanced, symmetrical and slightly uncomfortable (eg. sitting in a straight backed chair or lying on the floor) to lesson the chance of falling asleep.
2. Use a technique for physical relaxation. Muscles of the various parts of the body are relaxed in turn allowing them to feel "soft and loose ... heavy and warm ... deeply and completely ... just letting go". More feelings of relaxation encourage the mind to follow with a sense of calmness and peacefulness. "These are a few minutes just for you - nobody to please - nobody to care for ... nothing to bother you ... nothing to disturb you.
3. Adopt a passive attitude - not "meditate or bust!" The effort is in putting the time aside - not in meditating.
4. A period of mental stillness that leads the mind away from mundane matters.

Be warned about nimble minds, possible distractions (leave the phone off the hook and a note on the door) and allow interruptions to just disappear "like white clouds drifting across the blue sky". Don't expect every meditation to be a peak experience; there is some benefit in just sitting still. There are benefits in meditating even for a few minutes, better for 10-20 minutes once or twice a day! Losing sense of time some people enjoy meditating for much longer.

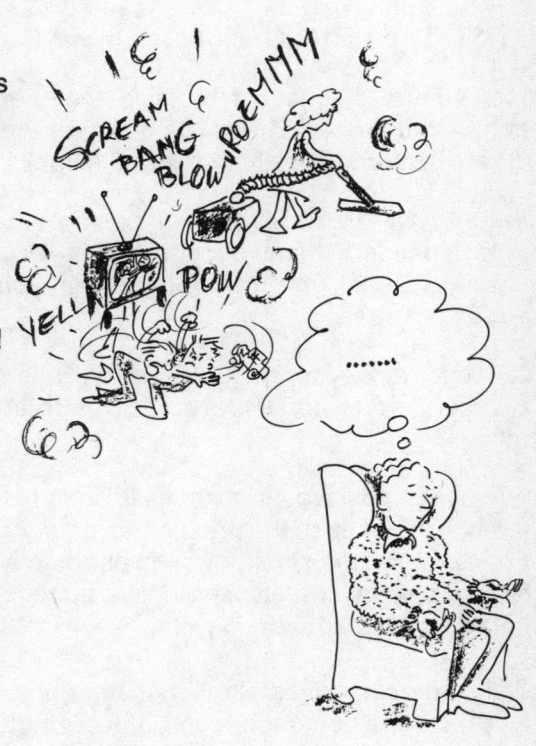

For some there is more to meditation than just health. Positive attitudes towards life and death develop as it becomes an experience that goes beyond the intellect and into the realm of spiritual awareness.

STEP OUT: THE TIME FOR ACTION

Cancer often stops people in their tracks. Three possibilities arise - some people prefer to deny it, others become depressed. The third possibility is to do something. Doing something demands change - it is time for action. We are not always responsible for what happens to us but we are responsible for how we respond to what happens. Cancer can be a reason for doing anything!

Use this opportunity to achieve a way of life that will give real and deep satisfaction that provides a genuine reason for being, and gives life the kind of meaning that makes you glad to get out of bed in the morning. Write the second edition of your life. Explore your best moments and set up life to include more of them. Celebrate what's right rather than look for what's wrong. There is something right within each of us that can be encouraged and activated, overcoming anything that may have restricted its perception or expression in the past. Find something that will make you enthusiastic about life. Start out in a small way, pace yourself, take pleasure in simple things, enjoy the scenery and be amazed at what is possible.

POSITIVE THINKING

Henry Ford of T model fame said "whether you think you can, or think you can't - you are right." Use the power of the mind to think positively and with creativity to resolve problems and establish new goals.

We all have the ability to think positively but sometimes it's too difficult and help is needed. Many people have mixed feelings about asking for help. Even if you ask you may not get what you want - but if you don't ask - the odds are worse.

Be clear about your goal. (Sharing it with someone else keeps you honest.) Be prepared to do whatever it takes to achieve that goal - then choose to enjoy it.

The use of positive affirmations is often helpful. These are statements about the future, made in the present, as if they had already happened in the past! For example, the smoker who is about to quit might repeat to himself "I am a happy, healthy non-smoker." Make up your own affirmation eg. "I am getting better and better every day."

Thinking positively is often difficult to both initiate and maintain and what is more, carries no guarantee - but the effort is worthwhile.

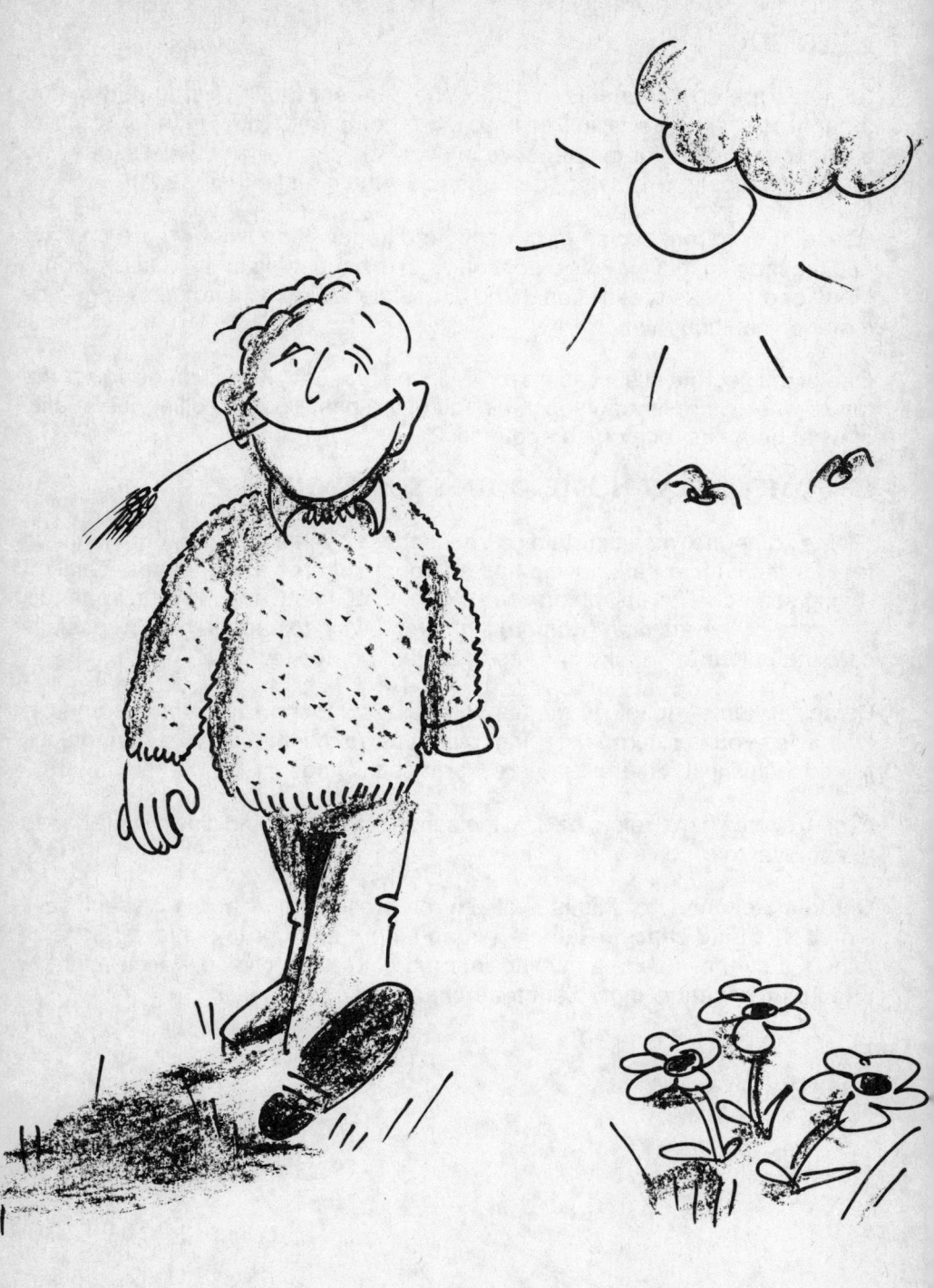

ATTITUDES

Attitudes are so important. Consider the different feeling generated by the thought that "my life is full of problems" compared with "my life is full of challenges". Look for the negative in every situation and you will surely find it. If life hands you a lemon, perhaps you should make lemonade!

Peace of mind must come from within and depends on what we are thinking and feeling and to a far less extent on what is happening in the outside world. Many of our ideas are irrational and cause disturbances if not challenged by more logical thoughts.

One of the secrets of success is to live in the present. Fear locates you in the future whereas resentment locates you in the past - both spoiling the quality of what happens today (see appendix 2).

BE SOMEONE, AT HOME, GOING SOMEWHERE

"Being someone" means retaining your sense of value as a person - no mean feat for the cancer patient who has no doubt suffered many losses. Think of "being someone" as just being you - a person of unique talents (see appendix 3), 'state-of-the-art' man (woman) kind, not having to depend on successfully carrying out certain tasks or roles to be that someone.

Being "at home" hopefully means you have someone to love and someone who loves you in return. Meaning to life has so much to do with harmonious relationships with others; they are worth cultivating.

"Going somewhere" refers back to the sense of purpose and discipline required to achieve your goals.

Unfortunately none of this is available on prescription - nor is it specifically aimed at curing cancer. Rather, it is an all out attempt to achieve peace of mind - a dynamic state achieved through conscious choice, which might in turn be an essential ingredient for a chance of cure.

USE YOUR IMAGINATION: WRITE YOUR OWN STORY

No great achievement is accomplished without a great dream preceding it.

PSYCHONEUROIMMUNOLOGY (MIND OVER MATTER)

Evaluation of psychological techniques such as meditation, mental imagery and hypnosis has become more scientific as the new medical specialty of psychoneuroimmunology researches what used to be labelled as placebo medicine i.e. really looking to see if "mind-over-matter" could be for real. This suggests that there is a link between body and mind - an idea which, in fact, has ancient origins.

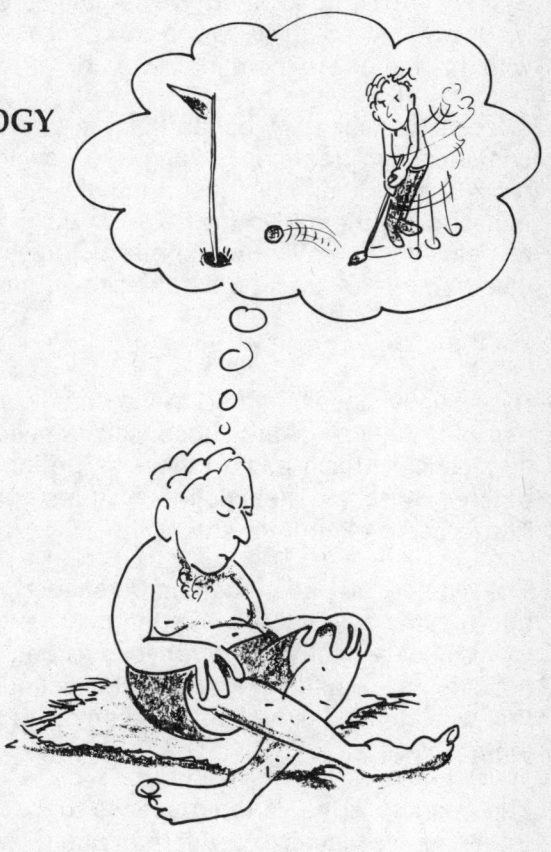

The new specialty proposes that the balance is between the mind, various hormones and the immune system. Disruptions in this balance have been shown to underly a number of diseases including cancer. It is possible that replacing negative thoughts with positive images using mental imagery or hypnosis may increase the chance of a healthy outcome.

MENTAL IMAGERY

Mental imagery or visualization is a technique used by serious sportsmen and women. In a relaxed state of mind they visualize the event for which they are training, taking it through to its successful completion. Before playing a shot, the golfer sees the ball driven straight down the middle of the fairway, chipped onto the green and putted straight into the hole. This doesn't guarantee a win but the chances of success are better than dwelling on a whole lot of negative thoughts about the outcome of their efforts.

Similar techniques have been recommended for cancer patients. In the Simonton's book "Getting Well Again" they suggest using imagery in the meditative state of mind, to see how effectively the cancer treatment is working, with the immune system mopping up.

Successful imagery requires that the cancer cells are seen to be weak and confused, the treatment strong and powerful. Any healthy cells damaged recover quickly and the vast army of white cells finishes off the cancer cells getting rid of them from the body. At the end of the imagery you see yourself as being healthy. Whether mental pictures need to be anatomically correct or can be more abstract probably does not matter.

HYPNOSIS

Hypnosis is closely related to the use of relaxation and imagery and makes use of the ability of the subconscious mind in the hypnotic state to take on suggestions which might otherwise be ignored. The hypnotic state can be entered by simple induction techniques not unlike those used in meditation. These can be learnt for self hypnosis.

The hypnotised patient can be persuaded to see himself as he would like to be - healthy competent and strong, living the kind of life he would most like to live. Some doctors favour hypnosis because they want the patient to believe that something real and significant is happening immediately and that with simple instruction they can make these important things happen themselves.

The problem is the varied response to these techniques by different people. Some people visualize better than others, some are better hypnotic subjects. It is possible therefore to feel a sense of failure, experiencing guilt and depression, adding to the level of tension. In spite of this there is sufficient evidence to support the use of psychological resources as a complementary treatment of cancer. Those who await final proof before being convinced may be like a contemporary of Aristotle's who decided never to say anything unless it was certainly true. It is said he ceased to talk and was confined to wagging his finger!

BE PRACTICAL: DIET, EXERCISE, PAIN CONTROL AND COPING DAY TO DAY

For a start being practical means recognizing that general advice about diet and exercise, pain control and coping might need to be varied according to the individual person and the stage of the illness. There are times when it won't be possible to stick to the Australian Dietary Guidelines for a healthy diet for well people or when the feelings of exhaustion and tiredness are so great that exercise is the last thing on your mind. Nevertheless what we eat makes a significant difference to the body's ability to resist disease and with exercise and other aspects of lifestyle is important in maintaining health.

DIET

Advocates of various diets for cancer provide the patient with a mountain of conflicting advice about what to eat, even though there is no diet which cures cancer.

However it is agreed that dietary fats are promoters of cancer. Fats lead to a sluggish circulation which is less efficient in carrying oxygen, thereby depriving tissues of adequate levels for healthy functioning. There is also evidence that a low fat diet may increase the activity of immune cells.

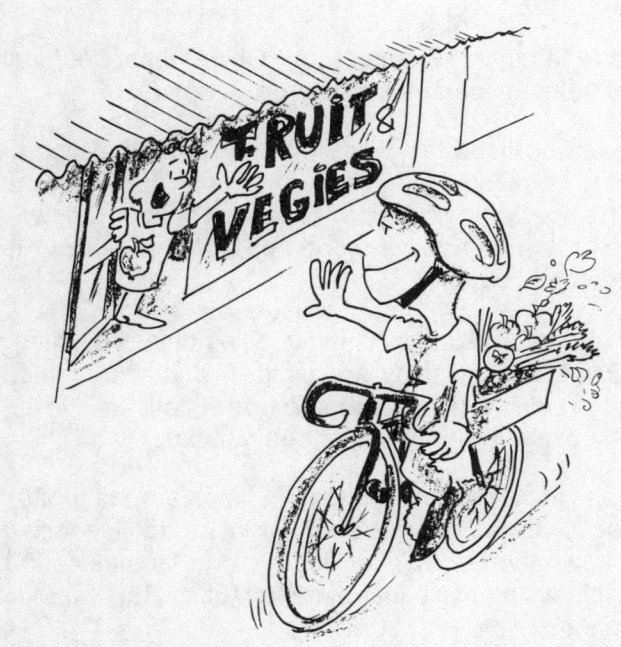

Any diet should therefore be low in fat and cholesterol (seeAppendix 7), contain a variety of foods to be nutritionally complete, be high in complex carbohydrates (present in vegetables, fruit, bread, cereals including oats, rice, pasta) and contain an adequate supply of protein (lean meat such as chicken, fish and low fat dairy products).

Eating should remain an enjoyable experience. A flexible and reasonable approach is necessary which may mean forgetting the traditional three meals a day. If there is poor appetite, nausea or weight loss, small frequent meals, favourite foods and high energy drinks can be helpful (Appendix 8). Blending fruit with low fat ice-cream is cool and moist, providing calories that slip down easily. Custards are often well tolerated. More detailed information is available from Anti Cancer Council publications.

VITAMIN AND MINERAL SUPPLEMENTS

Vitamins and minerals are often recommended (but not in huge doses) to guard against nutritional deficiencies and boost immune function especially through periods of hospitalization and treatment. Vitamins A, C and E and the mineral selenium are thought to mop up potentially cancer causing free radicals which are produced in the course of cell metabolism. As mentioned above excessive claims should not be made about the ability of diet to cure cancer but neither should its potential contribution be underplayed.

EXERCISE

"Man was made to move. (Woman too!) Only the hardiest individual should run the risk of being a spectator." George Sheehan.

Without exercise up goes the pulse rate, up goes the blood pressure - up goes everything you would like to go down, and down goes everything you would like to go up. Down goes your breathing capacity, down goes strength and endurance, down goes your mood and ability to relax. Fitness and well being fast become a memory.

By exercise is meant walking, swimming, bike riding or running depending on what you enjoy. Large muscles are used in rhythmic fashion at your own speed. Walking requires no special skills or athletic abilities. You can do it anytime, in any place, with or without companions.

To be worthwhile you need to exercise 3-4 times a week for 20-30 minutes. If gentle exercise is all that's possible try a mini trampoline for a walking action inside. Next down the list, is a rocking chair or isometrics in bed! Make no mistake - exercise is a physical and mental tonic. Tailor it to needs, abilities and circumstances.

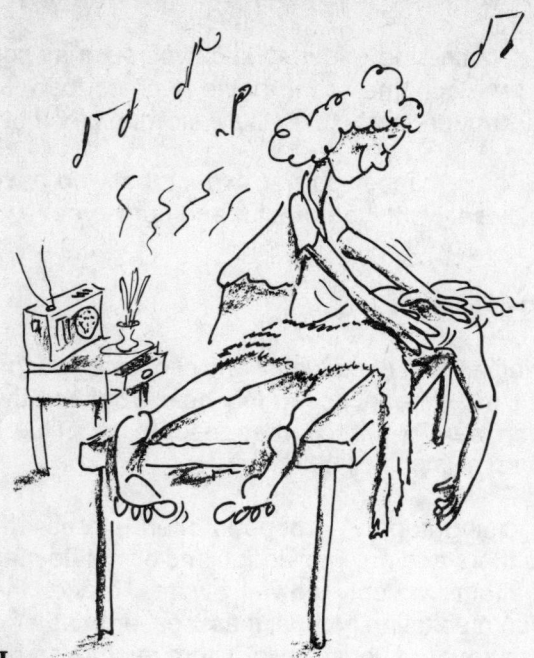

PAIN CONTROL

While not everyone with cancer suffers pain (in fact 30% do not) it is important to know that of those who do, the vast majority can expect pain relief and lead useful lives. There is more to pain than pain! That is, besides the physical sensation there is emotional suffering with pain and fear reinforcing each other. Anxiety, uncertainty, the various losses cancer patients face, social isolation,financial problems and spiritual concerns all aggravate pain. Dealing with these problems using meditation, hypnosis or counselling can all be helpful in pain management.

The cancer itself may need more treatment with surgery, radiotherapy or chemotherapy.

Medical regimes for pain control are usually simple beginning with tablets like panadol progressing to Codeine preparations and finally adding oral morphine if necessary. Other medications may be used as well eg. if the cancer is pressing on a nerve. The right medicine, in the right dose given regularly at the right time relieves most pain.

Morphine is usually started in liquid form changing later to long acting tablets. Taking morphine is not the big deal many people believe it to be. It does not mean approaching death (it just means severe pain), addiction is not a problem in this situation and larger doses can successfully be used if pain progresses.

Constipation is the main side effect so laxatives such as coloxyl with senna should be taken once codeine or morphine is prescribed. Morphine can be given in other ways eg. under the skin, if swallowing or vomiting is a problem.

Just because you have cancer do not expect that you have to put up with pain. By working closely with your doctor and nurse your cancer pain can be relieved.

COPING DAY TO DAY

Coping means living a life of high quality and choosing your priorities carefully. To achieve this it may mean accepting help from relatives and friends, community support services and other resources. This is not a sign of weakness nor an admission of failure.

Hesitancy about joining support groups is often expressed. Yet they offer companionship, understanding, knowledge and eliminate many of the barriers of which cancer patients are only too well aware. Through them there is often access to relaxation/meditation groups, massage, aromatherapy and volunteer assistance for both you and your family. There might also be the opportunity for you to help someone else through your own experiences.

Some or all of these avenues can be used to keep your pilot light burning through what could be difficult periods of personal adjustment and treatment.

STAY TUNED: FRIENDS AND FAMILY RELATIONSHIPS ARE VITAL

Cancer is a blow to every family it touches. How it is handled within the family depends to a large extent on the way that family has functioned in the past. Those who are used to sharing needs and feelings generally find it easier.

Cancer gives the opportunity to talk about many things that might otherwise have been left unsaid. Out of the fears, anxieties and frustrations may come a time of rapid growth for members of the family.

On the other hand new roles and demands may overload them and resentment can arise so easily. Conflicts may not be readily resolved and the equilibrium of the family might be threatened. There are no easy solutions but most people with cancer find the best choice is to share the diagnosis and give those closest to them the opportunity to offer support. Rather than trying to hide fears it is easier in the long run to confide them. In this way foundations of mutual understanding and trust are built. It pays to solve problems together rather than struggle with them separately. However, old difficulties will not just evaporate and it is important to choose the right time and place to talk.

Different people operate on different emotional timetables. Some are ready to talk while others are still coming to grips with the situation. They might prefer to remain withdrawn for the time being. No-one should be forced. Such clashing needs create the risk of people avoiding each other - "building walls instead of opening doors". Clues to when is a good time to talk to discuss the illness may be non-verbal body language with gestures and looks often conveying the real message. Unusual nervousness or spending more time than usual with someone may indicate a desire to talk but not knowing where to start. Talking may include expressing anger, fear and confusion and those closest to each other often bear the brunt of outbursts. It's okay to admit when you've had enough with a promise to return to the conversation later on.

There is a need to be prepared to be a good listener - being silent and perhaps feeling powerless. Good listening means paying attention, not thinking about other things or what you might say before hearing the whole message. It is especially important to stay tuned to the feelings behind the words and then check out that you are receiving the right message by restating what you have heard.

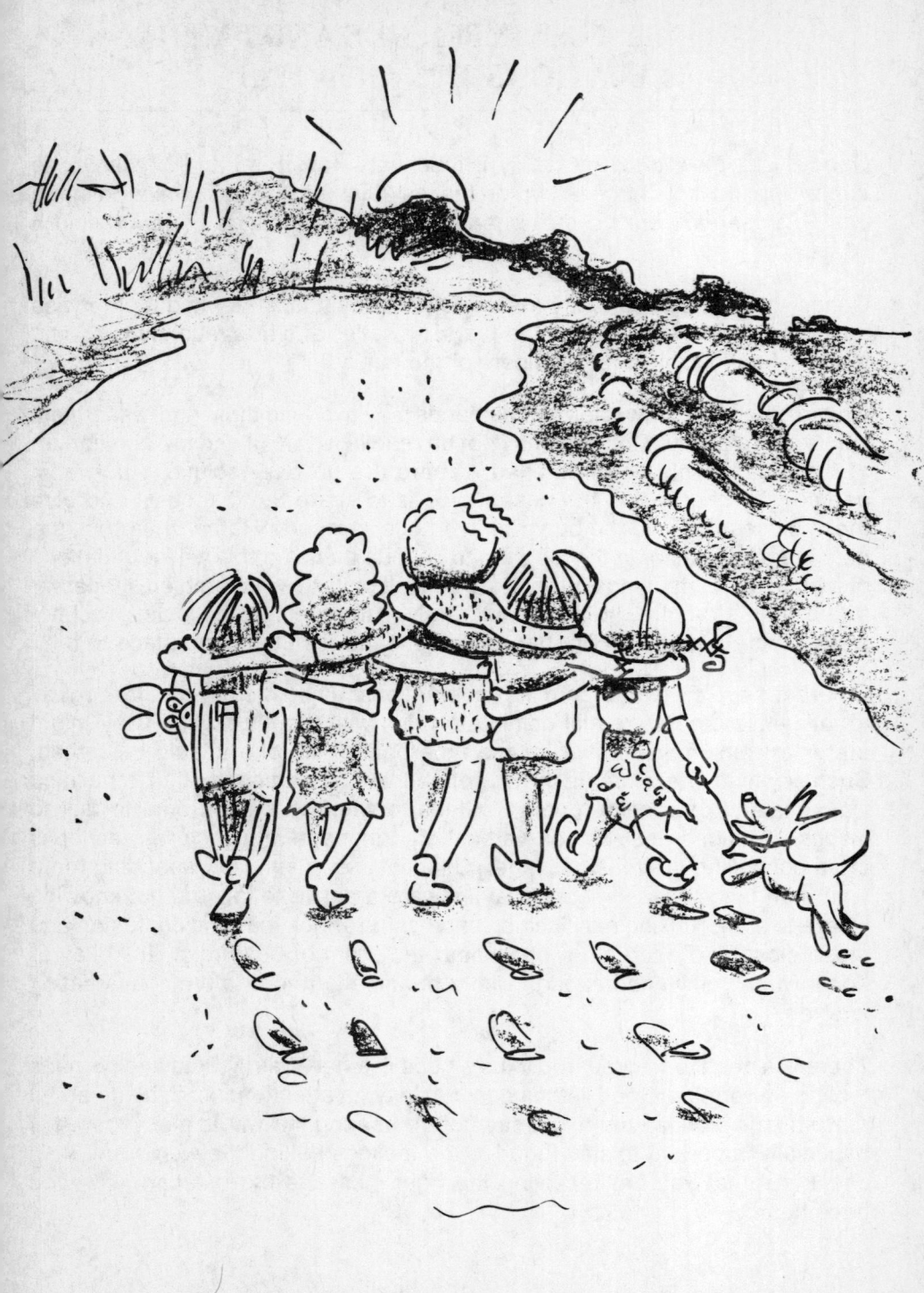

There are some common barriers to communication. False cheeriness "everything will be all right" and responses like "don't worry" or that's silly" deny people the opportunity to explore their feelings. Neither should you tell someone else "I know how you feel" - this is so unlikely!

Children should be given the opportunity to be included in discussions. They are sensitive to changed circumstances and need comfort, reassurance, affection, guidance and discipline when routines are disrupted.

The person with cancer needs family and friends as a constant in a changing world. Some friends may not call for a variety of reasons. Most will want to help but feel unsure about how to go about it. They may be waiting for some clue as to how to behave and be very grateful if there is something concrete they can do to show their continuing friendship. It might help to think of your requests for assistance as a way of letting friends feel useful. Lost friendships are one of the real heartbreaks that some people with cancer face. Answers are not easy but one person was quite philosophical; "I have some friends for when I am well and other friends when I am sick. I need them both."

FORGIVE: GETTING RID OF EXCESS BAGGAGE

There is no peace of mind with a troubled soul. Unfinished business - holding on to even the most righteous of indignations - ties people to painful pasts.

Achieving peace of mind means letting go of angry or defensive thoughts, judging thoughts, guilt, resentment, bitterness and hate - all excess baggage. None of these bring inner peace. The chain of attack and defence is endless. Anger is nothing more than attempts to make someone else feel guilty. No-one else can change our thoughts for us.

It might help to ask yourself the following question "Do you want to be happy or do you want to be right?" (G. Jampolsky). Being right does not necessarily lead to happiness. The argument may not be worth winning. The decision, after raising the above question, may be to let it go.

Judging thoughts do not bring peace of mind either. Our perception of others must be incomplete; we suffer from 'tunnel vision'. Would we be any different given their experience of life? Our sense of peace might also be destroyed by guilty thoughts. Self condemnation either leads to depressed feelings or a projection of the guilt onto someone else.

The antidote is forgiveness - starting with yourself and then extending it to others. Forgiveness is an essential ingredient in a loving relationship. Without it love becomes conditional, founded on getting and giving to get, on bargaining and trading "I will love you, if you ...." Unconditional love has no expectations or boundaries and sees the other person as either giving love or sending out a call for help requesting love.

Forgiveness is an exercise in our capacity to forget, relinquishing unhelpful trains of thought. It does not imply approval of someone else's behaviour or assuming a position of superiority to pardon sins. It sees beyond the more superficial motivation of an individual knowing that deep down they yearn for exactly the same as we do - peace of mind.

To experience forgiveness we need to offer it to others and then find that to give is to receive. Cross the bridge of forgiveness together and offer it to the world!

BE HAPPY: JUST FOR FUN?

"Life is a tragic comedy, a quirky combination of glory and grief, laughter and lows, joys and sorrows. Laughter lightens the load." R. Holden (1993)

There is not much that's less funny than being sick - and having cancer must be down the bottom of that list. Good grounds for being miserable and unhappy, mixed in with self pity. "Just leave me alone, I don't want to talk about it."

In 1964 Norman Cousins suffered from a rheumatoid condition involving his spine and joints that kept him flat on his back in pain. Although not medically trained, he researched the literature avidly to find plenty of evidence that negative emotions have negative effects on body chemistry. He wondered if positive emotions might just have positive effects. Could laughter enhance body chemistry? He decided to find out by watching funny movies, episodes of Candid Camera and the Marx Brothers' films. Ten minutes of laughter gave him a pain free sleep. This was the beginning of his recovery.

Thirty years later modern medicine is starting to prove the ancient theory that laughter is the best medicine. It is now known that endorphins (the body's own morphine like substances) are released and that the activity of the immune system is boosted.

So it would seem that being too busy to have fun is really serious.

There are good medical grounds to heed the bidding of the war time song "Pack up your troubles in your old kit bag and smile, smile, smile." With cancer on board there is an art to living happily, requiring certain basic beliefs to be complemented by practical strategies.

In "Laughter The Best Medicine", R. Holden (1993) makes the following observations:

> Happiness is an attitude which happens inside out - not outside in. It is something to be enjoyed along the way, not a destination, an essential lubricant for relationships which gives pleasure even when things are less than perfect. Laughter is a symbol of full, spontaneous, creative and peaceful living.
> To become happy it helps to act happy. Being silly is not so silly. Rather take care not to neglect so great a pleasure "A little nonsense now and then is relished by the wisest men."
> Donate a smile; give and you shall receive. "Laugh and the world laughs with you."

One essential ingredient for happiness is thankfulness. Make a list of things usually taken for granted for which you should be thankful. Share memories of happy occasions. Play games. "We do not stop playing because we are old. We grow old because we stop playing."

Begin a laughter library of books and videos. Is there something you could do right now to enhance your happiness? Don't wait - look at every area of your life. (Appendix 9) Be reminded of the need for enthusiastic living. Something which stirs you into action, which gives responsibility and meaning. Celebrate. Have a happy hour, a happy day, a happy new year.

And do it just for fun!

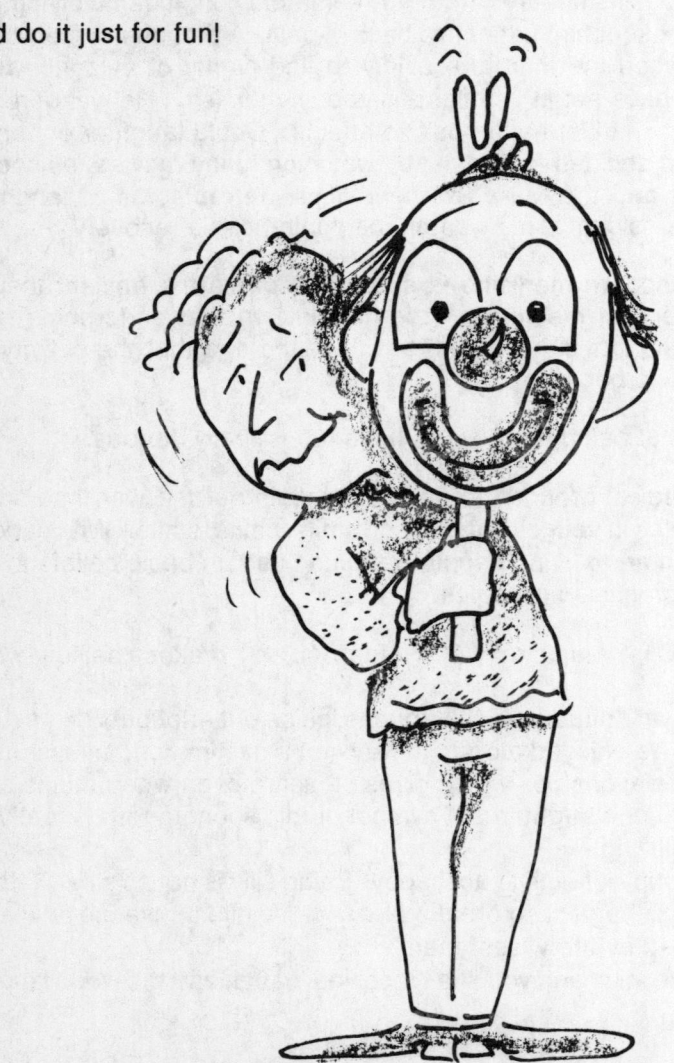

FIND THE MEANING OF LIFE: THE JOURNEY CONTINUES

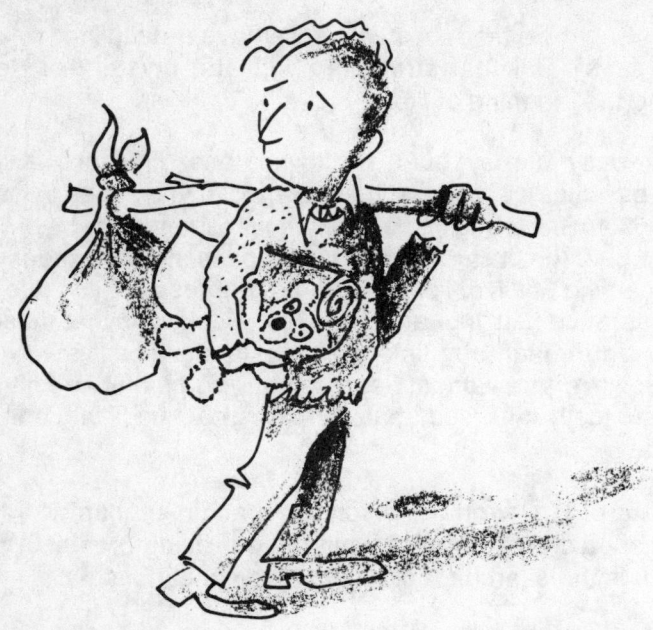

Life has a taste of mystery to it. No-one understands all its secrets and none of us really knows where we are going. According to Thomas Edison we don't even begin to understand 1% about 99% of anything.

There are some who search for pieces to the puzzle. But so many of us never really get started. Instead we hang on to some sense of immortality, knowing that one day everyone must die, yet behaving as if an exception will probably be made in our case!

George Sheehan, runner, writer and doctor who suffered from cancer of the prostate said that cancer is a blessing. It puts a sense of urgency into life, makes us see life as a gift and inspires us to think more about the human condition. Living becomes a matter of life and death and the search for meaning becomes paramount.

Many would argue that what gives meaning to life has more to do with how an individual stands in relation to his soul than to his physical frame. Scott Peck, author of "Further Along The Road Less Travelled" argues that everyone has a spiritual life, just as they have an unconscious, whether they like it or not. Some may try to avoid or ignore it but basically the puzzle is a spiritual one.

Spirituality may be found both inside and outside religious frameworks. Either way it is often through meditation that we come in touch with something deep inside. New insights can occur and changes in our lives result.

Peck agrees that we learn best when we have a deadline (what a wonderful word, he says) and that struggling with the mystery of death leads to discovering the meaning of life.

It is not an easy journey, but a worthwhile one. Elizabeth Kubler Ross, an American psychiatrist, defined the stages of dying in her pioneering work in the late 1960's. She found that people often respond to news of life threatening illness by denial (no, it can't be true), then pass through stages of anger (why me?), bargaining (if I live, I promise to ...), depression (it is true) and perhaps finally acceptance (it is true and it's O.K.). Peck says that these are also the stages we go through any time we make a significant step in our spiritual growth. However the work of depression is so painful and difficult (perhaps when we are justly criticised) that we may retreat back into denial, anger and bargaining.

The purpose of life, wrote Emerson, is to acquaint man with himself. That education should be interrupted only by our dying breath. We are here to learn and it is the search for meaning that is meaningful.

Growing spiritually is an ongoing process but according to Peck we cannot lose when we realize that everything that happens to us has been designed to teach us what we need to know on the journey. Progress is sometimes slow, sometimes rapid. If the meaning of life seems elusive, simply give meaning to life. To have a death worth dying you must have a life worth living. Many aspects of a person's life have spiritual significance but in particular relationships with families and friends have spiritual qualities. Through them we are able to add meaning to life.

Probably the puzzle will never be complete but perhaps there will be sufficient pieces to give a glimpse of the big picture. When we are on the right track, if only fleetingly, we realize it is only the philosophers and depressives who ask what is the meaning of life. When we are using ourselves in the way we are built for - we know.

DO IT IN STYLE: HOPE AND HEALING, LIVING AND DYING.

HOPE

"In the absence of certainty there is nothing wrong with hope." Bernie Siegel.

According to Ian Gawler, a survivor of widespread cancer, hope is the essential pre-requisite prior to the commencement of any healing program. Hopelessness arises out of a sense of powerlessness, fear and a denial of the possibilities. It leaves a trail of unhappiness and often premature death.

Facing reality and exploring the worst possibilities (often exaggerated by the mind) may leave room for a glimmer which leads onto hope for survival. There is no cancer from which someone has not been cured. It only has to happen once to be possible. Why not be the next?

However hope for survival is often driven by a fear of death and while there may be dramatic improvements in the short and medium term hope needs to progress to the next stage for a better long term outcome. Hope for a better future is based on the belief that there is a solution to current problems and this enables positive energies to be harnessed very effectively.

A sense of incompleteness and spiritual aspirations leads to the hope for a state of spiritual optimism. Progress to this stage is often slow requiring patience and resolve with support from other people, groups, books and tapes as well as personal practise in silence and meditation.

The final stage is hope to live contentedly in the present moment. The ability to cope with such ease in modern society is the ultimate in doing it in style.

HEALING

Healing has occurred when there is peace of mind. This distinguishes it from curing which does not necessarily lead to this point. In fact for those who go all out for a cure there is often a certain frenetic quality to their lives which does not lead to peace of mind. Healing goes beyond curing and may take place when curing is not an issue or has proved impossible.

However peace of mind is the one goal that creates the perfect environment for both healing and curing.

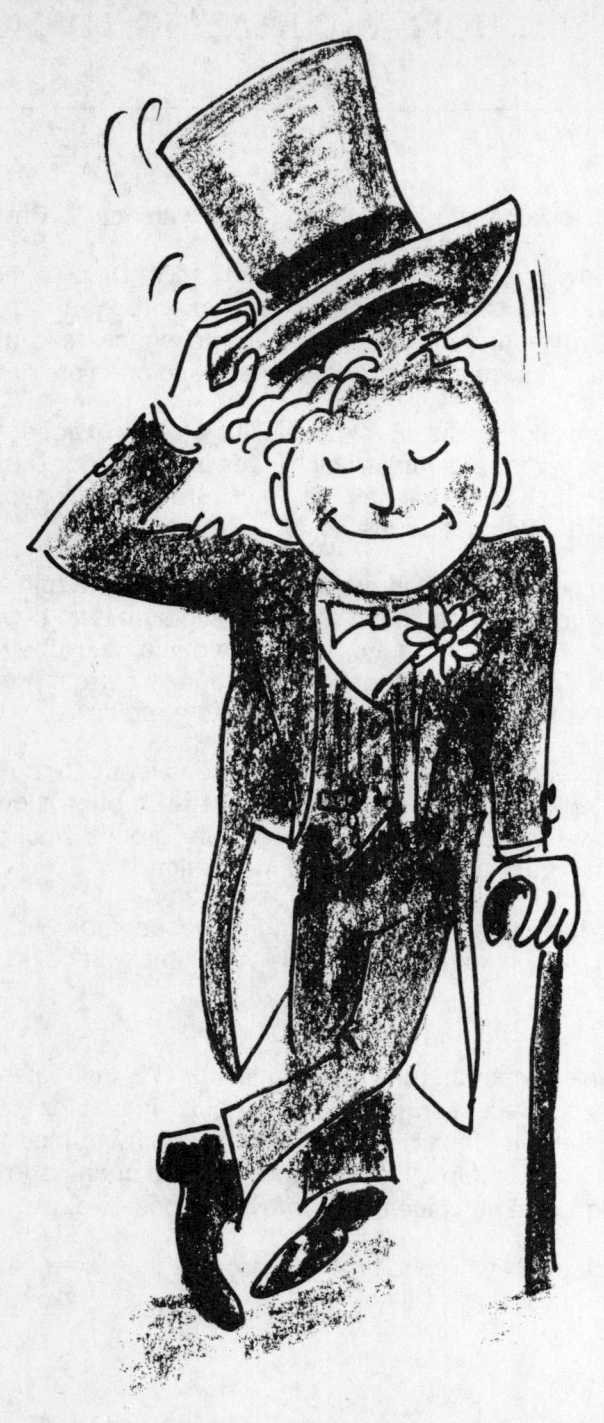

LIVING IN STYLE

This is reflected in the prayer "God grant me the serenity to accept the things I cannot change, courage to change the things I can and the wisdom to know the difference."

It may mean accepting limitations and adjusting priorities that reflect these. Maintain a purpose for living and express feelings. Don't aim to stay alive, but to live. A good quality of life means enjoying it, feeling challenged and fulfilled without the need to be perfect, having genuine satisfying relationships and not letting the little things that bring so much contentment slip by.

Remember that forgiveness is simply giving up all hope of a better past! All this means cultivating the art of taking time for ourselves. The need is to slow down, pause, breathe, be still, turn inward, listen. This is not something that society encourages - so like all things they are eventually done in style - requires practice, and more practice.

DYING IN STYLE

Sooner or later, whether from cancer or some unrelated cause the death rate becomes one per person. Eventually we all run out of loopholes and escape clauses. Preparing for the possibility of death does not interfere with the fight for life. In fact taking care of these things releases energy for living.

It is important to consider the likely sequel of events for the opportunity to have a sense of completeness, to put your affairs in order legally and financially and perhaps to plan a funeral. It is an opportunity to say what you've always wanted to say - write that letter, make that phone call, visit that friend.

Ensuring that you have the best medical care while dying is important - it may mean a different team from those treating you earlier on.

Give some thought to helping your loved ones with the grieving process. Take the opportunity to discuss your life history, the good and the bad, exciting times, major decisions, lessons learned and any regrets. How you die affects loved ones profoundly - it can be a time of growth and development. Eventually there is a need to let go of people and possessions.

There is a view that we are spiritual beings having a human experience and living on this planet in an effort to discover a higher state of consciousness. Death is the final pathway to that state of consciousness so we might as well do all we possibly can to leave in style!

The Wind Is Your Friend

It blew and blew and blew and blew,

Strong gusts scattered quite a few,

It was blowing quite a gale,

About force 9 on the measuring scale,

But we could handle it with ease,

To us it felt like just a breeze,

'Cos we are made of sterner stuff,

And any wind is just a puff!

E.F.

Look to this day!
for it is life,
the very life of life...
for yesterday is already
a dream,
and tomorrow is only
a vision:

But today, well lived,
makes every yesterday
a dream of happiness,
and every tomorrow a vision
of hope.

I'm Special

A POEM OF SELF WORTH

I'm special. In all the world there is nobody like me.
Since the beginning of time, there has never been another
person like me.

Nobody has my smile.
Nobody has my eyes, my nose, my hair, my hands,
my voice. I'm special.
Nobody anywhere has my tastes for food or music or art.
No one sees things just as I do.

In all of time, there has been no one who laughs like me,
no one who cries like me.
And what makes me laugh and cry will never provoke
identical laughter and tears from anybody else, ever.
No one reacts to any situation just as I would react.
I'm special.

No one in the universe can reach the quality of my
combinations of talents, ideas, abilities, and feelings.
Like a room full of musical instruments, some may
excel alone, but none can match the symphony sound
when all are played together.
I'm a symphony.
Through all of eternity no one will ever look, talk, think,
or do like me. I'm special, I'm rare.
I'm special.

And I'm beginning to realise it's no accident
that I'm special. I'm beginning to see God made
me special for a very special purpose.
He must have a job for me that no one else can do
as well as I. Out of all the billions of applicants,
only one is qualified, only one has the right
combination of what it takes.
That one is me.

TEN TWO LETTER WORDS

IF IT

IS TO

BE

IT IS

UP TO

ME

Happiness is like a butterfly

the more you chase it

the more it will elude you

but if you turn your attention

to other things

it comes and softly

sits on your shoulder

THE MIND IS

ITS OWN PLACE

AND

IN ITS OWN WAY CAN MAKE

A HELL OUT OF HEAVEN

AND

A HEAVEN OUT OF HELL

Suffering
is inevitable

Misery
is optional

THE FAT LIST

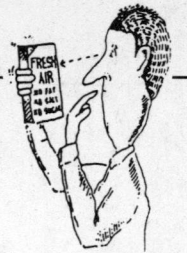

You may not have guessed how much fat is in many of the common foods that you eat. Check this list to find out where the fat in your diet is coming from.

Food	Fat(grams)	Food	Fat (grams)
Fruit & vegetables	0	Cheese (30g cheddar or cream)	10
Olives (5)	1	Cheese (100g cottage)	2-4
Avocado (½)	21	Cheese (30g light cream)	5
Coleslaw (10g tub purchased)	4	Cream (1 tablespoon)	8
Potato Salad (100g tub purchased)	6	Icecream (1 scoop)	5
Lentils (1 cup cooked)	0	Icecream (rich, 2 small scoops)	13
Soya Beans (1 cup cooked)	4	Milk (200ml regular)	8
Bread (2 slices)	1	Milk (200ml reduced fat)	4
Garlic Bread (2 slices)	9	Milk (200ml Shape or skim)	0
Rice & Pasta	0	Yoghurt (200g plain or fruit)	7
Breakfast cereal (average serve)	1	Yoghurt (small carton non-fat)	0
Toasted muesli (average serve)	12		
		Salad dressing (2 tablespoons)	16
Fish (average grilled fillet)	3	Mayonnaise (tablespoon)	16
Fish (1 piece 150g in batter)	24	Vegetable oils (1 tablespoon)	20
Salmon (100g canned)	8	Butter or margarine (1 tablespoon)	16
Tuna (100g canned in oil)	7	Rich fruit cake (average slice)	6
Tuna (canned in brine)	2	Cheesecake (average slice)	36
Sardines (100g canned in oil)	13	Apple pie (average slice)	19
Crab (100g fresh or canned)	1	Plain sweet biscuits 2 (25g)	4
Prawns (6 medium)	2	Sweet cream biscuits 2 (40g)	10
Lobster (½)	4	Chocolate biscuits 2 (32g)	9
Oysters (12)	1	Rye crispbread (2)	0
Mussels (6)	2	Sao (4)	6
		Hamburger (large)	31
Chicken (2 drumsticks with skin)	15	BBQ chicken (¼)	16
Chicken (1 breast fillet, 125g)	2	Meat pie or sausage roll (1)	24
Turkey (125g average serve)	3	Hot chips (250g average serve)	35
Rump Steak (200g grilled)	34	Pizza (½ medium)	16
Rump Steak (100g fat removed)	10	Chinese meals (average portion)	16
Beef mince (100g)	16	Fried rice (1 cup)	13
Veal (100g leg meat)	1	Crisps (small packet)	10
Lamb loin chops (2 grilled)	32	Popcorn (1 cup plain)	0
Pork Chop (1)	30	Nuts (50g)	23
Pork (100g lean new fashioned)	5	Chocolate (100g)	30
Rabbit (100g meat cooked)	2	Peanut Butter (1 tablespoon)	11
Ham (50g)	5	Jam (1 tablespoon)	0
Salami (50g)	19	Vegemite	0
Sausages (200g)	42		
Brains (1 set steamed)	11		

HIGH ENERGY DRINK SUPPLEMENTS

Often people find difficulty in trying to meet their nutritional requirements. The following drink recipes can be utilised as supplements both for and in between meal times. They are all very easy to prepare, the recipes can be altered accordingly, the only limitation being the makers imagination. The drinks can be made up and kept in the fridge throughout the day. You may prefer to pour small amounts into a glass frequently through the day or sit down and have a large glass 2-3 times during the day.

Apricot Lemon Crush

Apricot halves natural fruit juice	425g can
Natural yogurt	1 cup
Lemon juice	1 lemon
Honey	1 tble.sp
Wheatgerm	2 tble.sp
Ice	crushed
Glucodin	1 tble.sp

Blend all ingredients together

Banana Sustagen Drink

Milk	2 cups
Banana	one
Egg	one
Sustogen powder	3 dsrt.sp
Skim milk powder	1dsrt.sp
Glucodin	1 dsrt.sp
Ice	crushed

Vitamise all together

Egg Flip

1 egg	
Milk	1 cup
Vanilla syrup or essence	
Sugar	1 teasp.
Brandy	(optional)

*Vitamise all together,
strain, sprinkle with nutmeg if desired.*

Fruit Mix

Orange juice(or other fruit juice combination)	1 cup
Banana	one
Icecream and/or cream	1 scoop
Glucodin	1 dessertspoon
Ice	crushed

Vitamise all together

High Calorie Soup

Cream soup	55ml
Milk	55ml
Skim milk powder	1 tble.sp (6g)
Egg	one
Glucodin	1 teasp (2g)

Mix together thoroughly then vitamise. Heat slowly.

Fruit Shake

Milk	½ cup
Cream	1 tablespoon
Icecream	1 scoop
Stewed or soft fresh fruit	small serve
Skim milk powder	1 tablespoon
Glucodin	1 dessertspoon
Ice	crushed

Vitamise all together

Fruit Smoothy

Milk	1 cup
Banana	one (or other fruit)
Honey	1 tble.sp or sugar
Wheatgerm	1 tble.sp (if liked)
Icecream and/or cream	2 scoops
Ice	crushed

Vitamise all together, sprinkle with cinnamon if liked.

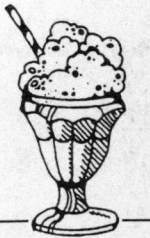

THE VITALITY QUESTIONNAIRE

This questionnaire is designed to highlight specific areas of your life that you may want to change. To give yourself a score from 1 - 10 it is necessary for you to imagine what it would be like to score 10.

The decision is yours if you want to achieve a different score. Establish your goal, do whatever it takes to achieve it and remember to enjoy it along the way.

	SCORE 1 TO 10	TOTAL
INTELLECTUAL LIFE		
1. Do you read books?	_____	
2. Are they mentally stimulating or informative?	_____	
3. Do you attend seminars, TAFE or other learning programs?	_____	
4. Are you well informed on current affairs, social, political, moral issues?	_____	
5. Do you attend exhibitions, concerts, visit galleries?	_____	
6. Do you practise art or craft?	_____	_____
SOCIAL LIFE		
1. Do you have many close friends (if 10 is a lot)?	_____	
2. How well does your closest friend know you?	_____	
3. Are you interested to meet new people?	_____	
4. Do you easily make friends?	_____	
5. Do you entertain or dine out with friends regularly?	_____	
6. Is your social life stimulating and energising?	_____	_____
EMOTIONAL LIFE		
1. How positive and pleasant are your emotions generally?	_____	
2. Do you easily resolve your negative emotions (fear, anxiety, resentment, loneliness)?	_____	

3. Are you aware at the time that your emotions are influencing your behaviour? _____

4. How well do you manage emotions that might tend to "carry you away" (excitement, delight, anger, grief)? _____

5. How free are you to express and accept feelings of affection? _____

6. How well do you handle embarrassment? _____ _____

PHYSICAL LIFE

1. How good is your relationship with your body? _____

2. Are you satisfied your normal diet is a reasonable one? _____

3. How appropriate is the exercise you give your body? _____

4. Do you frequently allow your body to relax? _____

5. How free is your body from the need for drugs (including alcohol, tobacco, prescribed medication, sleeping pills, etc.)? _____

6. How do you rate the energy level of your body, its vitality? _____ _____

SPIRITUAL LIFE

1. How strong is your belief in a supreme being? _____

2. How helpful to you is prayer, meditation? _____

3. Does your spiritual life promote your awareness of self-worth? _____

4. Does it bring you closer to others in love? _____

5. Do you feel your life is on course towards its ultimate purpose? _____ _____

FAMILY LIFE

1. How good is communication within your family? _____

2. Do you enjoy the time spent with your family? _____

3. How free are you to express your affection with your family? _____

4. Are arguments fairly and satisfactorily resolved? _____

5. Do you have joint projects, goals, play or outings? _____

6. Do you feel loved, as someone who really matters, by the other members of the family? _____   _____

LOVE LIFE

1. To what extent is your loving free from possessiveness or jealousy? _____

2. Is your expression of your affection for those you love free from self-consciousness, warm and spontaneous? _____

3. Are you comfortable receiving the affection of others? _____

4. Do you readily forgive and hold no resentment? _____

5. Are your relationships with those you love sharing and co-operative? _____

6. Do you love yourself appreciating your own worth? _____   _____

SEX LIFE

1. Do you have good communication on the subject with your partner? _____

2. Is intercourse an expression of mutual love between you? _____

3. Are you free from such disturbances as inhibitions, guilt, confusion, fear or other hang-ups? _____

4. How positively appreciative are you of your partner's expression? _____

5. Is love-making still as meaningful to you as ever? _____

6. Does your partner make you feel secure and appreciated? _____   _____

PROFESSIONAL LIFE

1. Are you satisfied this is the right career for you? _____

2. How adaptable would you be if this career were no longer possible or desirable? _____

3. Has your income been satisfactory and up to your expectations? _____

4. How eagerly do you anticipate the challenges and opportunities of your work? _____

5. How promising does the future look for further satisfaction or advancement? _____

6. How well are all your talents utilized in your present work? _____   _____

RECREATIONAL LIFE

1. Do you have a lot of different ways to play? _____

2. Do you allow time daily for recreation? _____

3. How much fun is the child in you allowed to have? _____

4. Is it easy for you to "act the goat" with friends? _____

5. Do you play with as much enthusiasm as you work? _____

6. How frequently do you allow yourself to do things "just for fun"? _____   _____

BE SIMPLE. BE KIND.

ATTEND TO YOUR INNER HEALTH AND HAPPINESS

(THIS MAY TAKE A LITTLE SELF DISCIPLINE!)

DO NOT STRAIN AFTER THE NEEDS OF LIFE -

IT IS SUFFICIENT TO BE QUIETLY ALERT AND AWARE OF THEM.

IN THIS WAY LIFE PROCEEDS MORE NATURALLY

AND EFFORTLESSLY.

LIFE IS HERE TO ENJOY.

From the Maharishi Code

The Rose

". . . it's the heart afraid of breaking,
that never learns to dance,
it's the dream afraid of waking
that never takes the chance,
it's the one who won't be taken,
who cannot seem to give,
and the soul afraid of dying,
that never learns to live . . "

Amanda McBroom

BIBLIOGRAPHY

1. About Cancer (1990) Anti Cancer Foundation, Adelaide S.A.
2. About Chemotherapy (1992) Anti Cancer Foundation, Adelaide S.A.
3. Barwood C. Secomb S. Meditating on Health Insurance Benefits, Australian Doctor Weekly
4. Brewster B. (1995) Physician Heal Thy Self, Mind Immunity and Health. Ed. I. Gawler, The Gawler Foundation
5. Byrski L. (1989) Facing Cancer: Searching for Solutions, Collins Dove, Blackburn Victoria
6. Cancer Treatment, Anti Cancer Council of Victoria Fact Sheet
7. Cousins N. (1979) Anatomy of an Illness, Bantam Books, New York
8. Dodd R. (1989) When you are Terminally Ill, Abingdon Press, Nashville
9. Doka K. (1993) Living with Life Threatening Illness, Lexington Books, New York
10. Eating Well, Anti Cancer Council of Victoria
11. Food for Faded Appetites, Anti Cancer Foundation, Adelaide S.A.
12. Fulgham R. (1991) "Uh-Oh", Grafton, London
13. Gawler I. (1984) You Can Conquer Cancer, Hill of Content, Melbourne
14. Gawler I. (1987) Peace of Mind, Hill of Content, Melbourne
15. Gawler I. (1995) The 5 Stages of Hope, Mind Immunity and Health. Ed. I. Gawler, The Gawler Foundation
16. Guex P. (1989) An Introduction to Psycho Oncology, Routledge, London
17. Hall C. (1982) Diagnosing Your Doctor, Cosmopolitan
18. Holden R. (1993) Laughter the Best Medicine, Thorsins, London
19. How to Communicate With Your Doctor, Living with Cancer Education Program, Anti Cancer Council of Victoria
20. Hunter M. (1987) Psych Yourself In, Seawalk Press, Canada
21. Jampolsky G. (1981) Love is Letting Go of Fear, Bantam Books, Toronto
22. Jampolsky G. (1983) Teach Only Love, Bantam Books, Toronto
23. Jampolsky G. (1985) Goodbye to Guilt, Bantam Books, Toronto
24. Johnson J., Klein L. (1988) I Can Cope, DCI Publishing, Minnesota

25. King P. (1992) <u>Quest for Life</u>, Random House, Australia
26. Le Shan L. (1984) <u>You Can Fight For Your Life</u>, Thorsons Publishers, Wellingborough, Northamptonshire
27. Le Shan L. (1989) <u>Cancer as a Turning Point</u>, Gateway Books, Bath
28. Lerner M. (1994) <u>Choices in Healing</u>, MIT Press, Cambridge, Massachusetts
29. Manion G. <u>The Vitality Questionnaire</u>, Bundeena, N.S.W.
30. National Cancer Institute (1985) <u>Taking Time</u>, NIH Publication Bethesda
31. <u>Patient Guide to Radiotherapy</u>, Peter MacCallum Cancer Institute
32. Reynolds T. (1987) <u>Your Cancer, Your Life</u>, Greenhouse Publications, Richmond, Vic
33. Rinpoche S. (1992) <u>The Tibetan Book of Living and Dying</u>, Harper, San Francisco
34. Scott Peck M. (1993) <u>Further Along the Road Less Travelled</u>, Simon and Schuster, New York
35. Sheehan G. (1979) <u>Running and Being</u>, Horowitz Publications, Hong Kong
36. Sheehan G. (1987) <u>Cancer and the Gift of Life</u>, The Physician and Sports Medicine Vol. 15 No. 12
37. Simonton O., Simonton S., Creighton J. (1978) <u>Getting Well Again</u>, Bantam Books, New York
38. Spiegel D. (1993) <u>Living Beyond Limits</u>, Times Books, New York
39. Templestowe V. (1991) <u>Let's Get The Fear Out Of Cancer</u>, Gateway Books, Bath
40. Van Bommel H. (1987) <u>Choices</u>, N.C. Press, Toronto
41. Wilkie A. (1993) <u>Having Cancer and How to Live With It</u>, Hodder & Stroughton, London
42. Gawler G. (1995) <u>Women of Silence</u>: The Emotional Healing of Breast Cancer. Hill of Content, Melbourne

ACKNOWLEDGEMENTS

This booklet has grown out of my involvement with the Living with Cancer Education Program of the Anti Cancer Council of Victoria, and with what was the Australian Cancer Patients Foundation, now the Gawler Foundation.

In his book "Uh-Oh", Robert Fulgham says that even the man who invented essays in the 16th Century - Michel Eyquem de Montaigne - insisted that his ideas and concerns were not original.

> "It might well be said of me that here I have merely made up a bunch of other Men's flowers and have brought nothing of my own but the string that ties them together in a bunch, which I gladly offer to you."

And so it is with this booklet. (I couldn't have said it better myself!) Each of the Authors mentioned in the bibliography has contributed significantly.

For helping me in the choice of material included I am grateful to those people with cancer and their families who have attended education groups in Warrnambool over the last ten years.

Thanks are also due to Boré Hoekstra for his illustrations that lighten the text, and to Pam Clark for her typing skills and enthusiasm.

Dr Eric Fairbank
Director of Palliative Care
Warrnambool & District Base Hospital